Autumn of Life

Autumn of Life

A Guide to Aging and Dying

Joseph Marino RN BSN

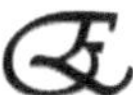

Strategic Book Publishing and Rights Co.

Strategic Book Publishing & Rights Co., LLC
USA | Singapore
www.sbpra.net

For information about special discounts for bulk purchases, please contact Strategic Book Publishing and Rights Co. Special Sales, at bookorder@sbpra.net.

ISBN: 978-1-68235-270-0

Dedication

To my dad, Hugo "Babe" Marino, who died way too soon and alone.

To my mom, Diane, my wife, brothers and sisters, my daughter and her husband, and my five grandkids.

Most of all, to all those patients and families that I served over the years. May those who have passed rest in peace.

And to a special friend and colleague, JoAnne Simonian, RN, who passed before this book was finished. She helped me understand the true meaning of death and dying. RIP, JoAnne.

Acknowledgments

I thank Lisa Foster, PT, for taking time out of her busy life to edit this manuscript, give me constructive criticism, and encourage me to keep going on this book. Thank you, Lisa.

Table of Contents

Preface

I have worked in the field of death and dying for over thirteen years as a gerontologist/hospice nurse and have studied the past as an anthropologist. I have lectured on social anthropology, death and dying, law and ethics in healthcare, and was a member of several ethics committees. Combining anthropology and healthcare has given me a unique understanding of aging and death and dying, not only of early humanity but modern humans as well. In putting together this book, my goal is to give this generation and the next information on what I believe are the important aspects of this area and what I have seen over the years.

This book is a guide to beginning students studying humankind in some form or another, including psychology, anthropology, sociology, or teachers or anyone interested in aging, and death and dying. More importantly, it's aimed at future nurses, medical students, medical social workers, clergy, and caregivers serving the aging and dying. As experienced caregivers, nurses, and social workers phase out and retire, younger staff need to replace them, and they need to have the knowledge to carry on with this work. When medical personnel have this knowledge, they teach the caregivers, which are usually families and friends, in how to care for that person that is failing in health. When these people have proper knowledge there is less panic among family, and the person that is dying dies peacefully in their own setting, not in a hospital bed or alone.

It's important to point out that not all views are compatible. Ideas and views of the world develop over time. The way one grew up, one's environment, influences, and the media shape one's views of different cultures or ethnic groups. However, the one thing that stays constant is death, the process, and how family and friends view and embrace it.

One of the purposes of this book is to open minds and hearts to a new way of understanding and feeling about aging, death, and the dying process. Most people are afraid of death. They will ignore it or deny it, shy away from it, and not talk about it, however, death should be embraced as part of the life process and to celebrate a person's life as they knew it.

The following information is meant to increase your awareness of aging, the dying process, and the issues surrounding it, along with the stigma and realities.

Death is each person's own experience. One doesn't have to die alone, but one does have to do it in their own way. Part of life is dying and finding one's own path to the way one wants to live and die. There is no "best" way to die. No one person's or society's way is better than another's.

All things that live die—plants, animals, and cells. However, humans are the only ones to memorialize their dead. Families use ceremonies, lay items in the grave of the deceased, and have wakes to honor the dead. To think about it and to dwell on it can hasten the process. The goal is to live your life as fully as possible. Enjoy the moments and the journey that life unfolds for you, and when it is time to die you can do it your way, quoting Frank Sinatra's "My Way." *(Paul Anka, 1969)*

And now, the end is near
And so I face the final curtain
My friend, I'll say it clear

I'll state my case of which I'm certain
I've lived a life that's full
I traveled each and every highway
And more, much more than this
I did it my way.

Prologue

To a child, the world is new and exciting. Life is full of mystery, fun, and imagination; wonderment is the focus.

To a teenager, the world becomes intriguing, with new friends, new relationships, new challenges, and learning to grow both mentally and physically.

To an adult, the world has changed, with responsibilities, family, happiness, loss, and fear of the unknown.

To the elderly, responsibilities lessen, losses increase, sadness becomes a way of life, and the unknown rears its ugly head and waits no more.

Chapter 1

Culture: Defining and Understanding

To understand death and dying, one needs a basic understanding of cultures, ethnic groups, and how people view them. Everyone has some basic culture or ethnic background as they see life in their own terms and what they learned growing up. This section sets the stage for the rest of the book. Culture is what drives most of us in our daily lives, and understanding culture will help us understand how to engage the aging person.

Let's step back to antiquity. Archaeological evidence shows that Neanderthals were the first early humans to bury their dead. Remains were found with a bison leg on the chest, and the grave was filled with broken animal bones, pollen from flowers, and flint tools. These artifacts were viewed as provisions for the long trip to the afterlife. Throughout history, primitive people buried their dead with food, weapons, and other goods representing provisions for the trip to the afterlife or spirit world. With this evidence, we can safely assume that these communities and families practiced the art of taking care of the dying and honoring the dead.

Does that differ today in modern times? No, not really, families bury their dead with items that the deceased was close to. Also, a person can request to be buried in their favorite car, in their favorite clothes, and kids are buried with toys and dolls.

So what does this mean? Basically, the same thought process is going on today as in the distant past; these items are there to keep the spirit company in its journey to the afterlife.

How does culture play a role in people's lives, especially when they are critically ill and dying? First, we have to understand what the definition of culture is.

There are a number of definitions. Here's a simple one:

Culture is that complex whole which includes knowledge, behaviors, art, beliefs, attitudes, morals, laws, values, ideals, and any other capabilities and habits acquired by humans as a member of society. It is the primary nonbiological means by which human societies adapt to and accommodate their environment. It refers to the innumerable aspect of life.

Culture embraces language, dietary habits, health practices, expressions of spirituality, and ways of celebrating. Culture also enforces the standards (rules) established by the group based on the values and beliefs of the group. Cultural differences among ethnic groups may include family organization, personal space, communication, beliefs about health, illness, healthcare practices, religions, and traditions.

How does one describe a culture? When anthropologists look at a culture, they focus on the customary behaviors rather than individual ones. There are also constraints which must be dealt with: direct constraints use force to ensure conformity, and indirect constraints discourage nonconformity by ridicule or social isolation. There are also adaptive traits, which are those that enhance the chances that the culture will survive in its particular environment. One term that anthropologists use to define culture is cultural relativism, which has a twofold meaning. One is the idea that one must not judge other cultures using his or her own culture as a criterion or basis; no culture is better or worse than any other culture, but each is relative to itself. Every culture is simply different, no better or worse than any other. The opposite of cultural relativism is "Noble Savage," the romanticizing of another culture. The problem with cultural relativism is that we judge people and cultures by our own set of criteria. Every country in the world has its own unique culture, except the US, which is a conglomeration of other cultures.

Within a culture are feelings that the individual culture is superior to other cultures, as is noticed throughout history with religious wars, genocide, and crusades. Each society felt that they were the superior society, and all others were inferior. There are modern-day examples. One was the Holocaust. Not only were Jews persecuted, but anyone not pledging allegiance to the Nazi regime was put in concentration camps and put to death.

To understand these differences, there are some important definitions. *(Ember & Ember, 1990)*

Stereotype: Forming specific beliefs about groups of people. These beliefs become rigid and are based on generalizations.

Ethnocentric: Characterized by or based on the attitude that one's own group is superior.

Ethnocentrism: Judging another culture solely by the values and standards of one's own culture.

Ethnicity: Refers to special groups within a race as defined by national origin or culture. Members of an ethnic group share common traits, including heritage, national origin, social customs, and language.

Society: A group of people who occupy a specific locality and who share a common language and cultural traditions.

Social structure: The relationship of groups within a society that hold it together.

Subculture: A distinctive set of standards and behavior patterns by which a group within a larger society operates. An example is the Amish, who have their own way of life, control their own schools, instill Amish values in their children, dress in one style, and have no electricity or motorized vehicles.

Enculturation: The process by which a society's culture is transmitted from one generation to the next. Culture is learned rather than inherited; one grows up with it. This is different than traditions, which are within the family.

Culture includes thoughts (worldliness) and behaviors (rituals), learned by tradition and wisdom vs. inherited (DNA). Culture is learned as a whole, with systems integrated with beliefs and behaviors and shared by individuals.

America's view of Death and Dying:

Let's explore how Americans view death and dying. America is a melting pot of other cultures. For the most part, America was settled by immigrants from England who brought their values, religions, and customs with them. So why do Americans deny death? We put a psychological block on it, we don't want to admit it, we ignore it, pretend it is not there, dismiss it—whatever terms you want to use.

The physician takes a Hippocratic oath by which they are bound to do no harm and treat the sick to the best of their ability. Based on this oath, the physician is to sustain life as long as possible, and that is what we come to accept, and it's also where people don't understand the limits of medical technology. Because of this oath, physicians are in a bind medically and ethically when treating the sick and injured. Medical technology is growing so fast that they are in a quandary as to when to let go or tell the family that there is no more that can be done. There have been a number of instances where a person is starting the active phase of dying (which we will get into in later chapters), and off to the hospital they go, families hoping for miracles where there are none.

In this country, we are so entangled in material wealth that we can't see the forest for the trees. We place more meaning on material wealth than we do on what life is supposed to be about. Look around at all the gadgets and toys that are being produced. Each year there is a new version of a phone, or the latest, greatest electronic gadgets, which are getting smaller and thinner each year. There is a saying that has been going around, "Those who die with the most toys win." Americans are creatures of comfort. We want what will keep us happy, so we can ignore the outside world and what is happening around us. This also applies to their families and friends when they age and die. Americans lack the familiarity of death. They are separated from their elders by distance, and in some cases by choice, and they don't see them aging and dying, and only come for the funeral. The care of the aging and dying are in the hands of the medical community and caregivers that are strangers to them vs. the family caring for their loved ones. So, for the most part, there is a breakdown in the family unit. Americans would rather put their loved ones in residential community homes, group homes, assisted living facilities, or nursing homes. We intellectualize death rather than experience it, and we don't care for our loved ones when they die; we leave it to the morticians. We lack control over it, or it is beyond our control, so we ignore it. Death is impersonal to Americans because we are so far removed from it that we have no idea how to deal with it.

Denial in the American culture regarding death is seen more in the modern era, about the early 1900s to the present. Prior to this, as America was growing, there were still a lot of small towns. We didn't have the medical technology we do today, so families still took care of their elderly family members. They cared for them in illness and in the dying phase, and when they died, they treated the body up to the point of the funeral. They had no fear of touching the corpse, cleaning it, dressing it, and getting it ready for burial.

In today's society, there is a lack of preparation when someone dies. People are sometimes caught off guard, saying that they weren't expecting it or just didn't know. There is anxiety or fear in touching a corpse; cosmetics make a corpse look lifelike. Americans spend all kinds of money to embalm the person, for caskets, metal vaults to keep the corpse from decaying. Today there is a new trend of drive-up funerals—drive up, pay your last respects, and leave. Wakes are shorter, and families will hide the children from viewing the body. Funeral homes close early in the evening, so visitations are cut short and funerals quickened. No sooner is the corpse laid out then they are driving it to the cemetery for burial, giving the family really no time for the mourning process. There is little time to grieve, and grieving is usually not public. Even the tombstones now are flat, with only the name, date of birth, and date of death on it.

This is the now society. We want things now, fast, and don't want to wait for anything. Funerals and mourning cut into Americans' time. Companies only give three days off, and that has to be for an immediate family member, and if you are full-time. If not, you have to take off on your own time. With the advent of the Internet, funeral homes are starting to show the funeral over the Internet for families and friends that are away and can't make it physically to the funeral.

There are still some traditions that are followed here in America. There are cities and towns that hold parties at the wake and following a funeral. For example, in New Orleans, they have a unique way of celebrating life and death that arose from African spiritual tradition, French musical traditions, and

African American cultural influences. It is a jazz funeral, which begins with a march of family and friends to the cemetery with somber music honoring the dead. Once the funeral has concluded, the procession marches back home and the music is very loud and upbeat with dancing, and onlookers may join in for the celebration of the life.

Police and fire departments have their own funeral processions. You may have seen this, where the casket is placed on the fire truck draped with an American flag, and personnel from both police and fire proceed and follow this truck. They will have two ladder trucks, with both ladders raised at the cemetery and crossed, where the procession will proceed underneath. These services will involve the honor guard from the police and/or fire department. Canada has the same type of funeral, and some representatives from other countries will attend to honor the fallen comrade.

Defining different cultures' practices of honoring their dead is a book in itself. For purposes of this book, to understand aging, death and dying, one must have a basic understanding of what culture is all about. When one has that, one will appreciate people as they get older.

Chapter 2

Physiology: Process of Aging and Dying

In America we live in an aging society, a society in which baby boomers are getting to retirement age. This will put a strain on our society to care for them.

A term that is normally used for aging is senescence, which means to grow old. It follows that as people get older there are functional and biological changes.

What happens when you die? Well, dying is basically the biological process in which the body's function slows down to a point where the slowing of the blood flow inhibits the organs to function properly, eventually shutting the body down. We can say in general terms that by the time you are twenty-five or so, your body is dying. Blood cells carry oxygen and nutrients throughout the body, so as aging occurs, the bone marrow that makes the blood cells don't make as many as when you were younger. There are many theories to the aging process, some of these are immunity theory, DNA crosslink theory, free radical theory, stress theory, etc. *(Matteson, 1988)*

What we do know is that aging is a complex phenomenon. All species age at different rates, and different factors influence the speeding up or slowing down of this process.

Some definitions to explore:

Lifespan is the length of life of an individual or the average length of life in a population or species. *(Mosby Dictionary, 2013)*

Life expectancy is the probable number of years a person will live after a given age, as determined by mortality rates in a specific geographic area. It may be individually qualified by the person's condition or race, sex, age, or other demographic factors. *(Mosby Dictionary, 2013)*

Remember that aging, death, and dying cross all lines of culture, ethnic groups, races, and religions. It is common to all living species on earth. So now that we got that out of the way, let's explore this dying process a little deeper. We live in a society that marvels in its accomplishments to keep a person alive. Diseases killed or crippled millions of people a couple of centuries ago (the Black Plague or the crippling effects of polio in the early twentieth century). We now have antibiotics and cures for such diseases. Medical technology is growing at a rapid rate. There's genetic engineering of drugs and cells, organ transplants, pacemakers, AICD (implantable defibrillators), cancer-fighting drugs, which twenty years ago didn't exist, and more are coming out every year. As a society we fight, scratch, claw our way from death's door. There are health products that claim will shave years off of your age and make you look young again, plastic surgery, Botox (which a derivate of the botulinum toxin); we are all looking for the fountain of youth.

However, out of all these technological advances, we still die. Our bodies just give up; there is only so much we can do to keep alive. There are still diseases out there that will kill us, for example, ALS (amyotrophic lateral sclerosis, commonly known as Lou Gehrig's disease), which is a devastating neuromuscular disease attacking the nerve cells in the brain and spinal cord, shutting down the motor neuron, causing paralysis and death. Even with this disease, we can keep the body functioning with a respirator and a computer so that the person can communicate with the outside world. (We will get into the ethical issues in another chapter.) With Parkinson's disease, Alzheimer's, multiple scleroses, muscular dystrophy, and a long list of many other diseases, we do not have cures, and having one of these diseases is basically a death sentence.

This leads us into the functionality of the dying process. What happens to the body when we die? It depends on the type of disease we have. For example, if a patient has CHF (chronic heart failure) the atrium and ventricles of the heart don't work the way they should. The physiology of the heart is that the unoxygenated blood coming from the veins in the body goes into the right atrium, which pumps the blood into the right ventricle, where a valve shuts behind it, then the right ventricle pumps the blood out through the pulmonary artery to the lungs, where the lungs oxygenate the blood by exchanging the PO2 (partial pressure of oxygen), with the PCO2 (partial pressure of carbon dioxide). The oxygenated blood then goes through the pulmonary vein back to the left atrium, then is pumped into the left ventricle, where another valve closes (these valves prevent a backup of the blood) from there the blood is pumped through the aorta back into the body. Now with CHF, these chambers and/or valves not working correctly can make the fluid back up into the body where you will see edema in the legs, and if not taken care of, fluid will build up in the lungs. *(Berkowitz, 2007)*

Neuromuscular diseases affect the nerves in the brain and spinal cord, shutting down the motor neurons, leaving one paralyzed. The person will then die of complications related to this disease, often pneumonia. What if we don't have those dreaded diseases, and we are fortunate enough to live to our eighties or nineties? Our bodies slow down, things just get, old like the parts of a car that wear out, and then we replace them.

Not so easy with the human body. Our intake of fluid and food decreases, our metabolism changes, we tire easily, our eyes don't see as well, our minds slow down, forgetting words that used to come easily to us. As the person slowly fails, there is a myriad of things that the body goes through. Dying and death is a simple but complicated process. Simple as the family or loved ones look on, but complicated for the person going through the dying process.

Let's talk about this dying process. Being a hospice nurse for over thirteen years, the author has dealt with hundreds of deaths and counseled many families through this process. Again, people die in their own time and their own way. Some patients want their family and loved ones around, and others will wait until they leave the room so as not to let them see them die. This sometimes brings guilt to the families. However, this is what the dying person wanted. This person has control and will choose the time they die. Some people wait until after the holidays, then die, or after a special occasion, so as to not ruin it for their families.

Let me give you examples of what I mean. A patient of mine was in the process of dying; her body was giving out, with no one specific disease. She lived in a nursing home, and her family would visit every day and spend hours with her. One day as I was working with another family, I saw this family leave. They stopped and said to me that they were going to have some lunch, clean up, and come back, to which I said that I probably would still be here. The family left and a few minutes later the aide for that floor went into the room to check on her. She came back and told me that she had died. I went in and checked her, then pronounced her death. I called the family and told them what had happened and to return. When they arrived, we spoke, and they said that they just left to get some rest and would return. I told them that she chose that time to pass away, as she did not want them to see her die. They were sad but relieved as she passed peacefully and on her own time.

Another story, more personal to me, was when my grandmother died. She was living with my aunt in Cleveland. My grandmother was in perfect health and ninety-six years old. The routine was that every night my aunt would bring my grandmother to the bathroom and then lay her down. Being the devoted Catholic she was, she made the sign of the cross and went to sleep. One night, as my aunt described, she was following the same routine, but she made the sign of the cross three times and never woke up the next morning.

One more story: I was seeing some patients in a nursing home, and as I walked down the hall, one of my patients that I happened not to be seeing that day came out and stopped me. We talked and then she said, "I am very grateful for knowing you and taking good care of me, however, I will not be here tomorrow." I really wasn't sure what she meant by the statement, but I acknowledged her and went about my day. The next day I came to see her, and the nurse that worked there told me she had died early that morning. As many patients that I have seen die, each had their own story to tell. Why am I telling you these stories? That although the death of a loved one is hard, scary, sad, one must cherish them while they are alive and listen to their story.

Let's talk about the physiology of the dying process. Death is a basic element of life; along with the emotional factors, there are physiological factors that control this.

Preparing for death physically: When a patient enters the final stages of the dying process, two different dynamics are at work, which are closely interrelated and interdependent. The two dynamics are physical and emotional/spiritual in nature. On the physical plane, the body begins the final process of shutting down, which will end when all the physical systems cease to function. Usually this is an orderly and undramatic progressive series of physical changes, which are not medical emergencies requiring invasive interventions. These physical changes are a normal, natural way in which the body prepares itself to stop, and the most appropriate kinds of responses are comfort-enhancing measures.

On the emotional-spiritual-mental plane, the spirit of the dying person begins the final process of release from the body, its immediate environment, and all attachments. This release also tends to follow its own priorities, which may include the resolution of whatever is unfinished of a practical nature and reception of permission to let go from family members. These events are the normal, natural way in which the spirit prepares to move from this existence into the next dimension of life. The most appropriate kinds of responses to the emotional-spiritual-mental changes are those which support and encourage this release and transition. When a person's body is ready and wanting to stop, but the person is still unresolved or unreconciled over some important issue or with some significant relationship, he or she may tend to linger in order to finish whatever needs finishing, even though he or she may be uncomfortable or debilitated. On the other hand, if a person is emotionally-spiritually-mentally resolved and ready for this release, but his or her body has not completed its final physical shutdown, the person will continue to live until that shutdown process ceases.

The experience we call death occurs when the body completes its natural process of shutting down, and when the spirit completes its natural process of reconciling and finishing. These two processes need to happen in a way appropriate and unique to the values, beliefs, and lifestyle of the dying person. The emotional-spiritual-mental and physical signs and symptoms of impending death, which follow, are offered to help you understand the natural kinds of things that may happen and how you can respond appropriately. Not all of these signs and symptoms will occur with every person, nor will they occur in this particular sequence. Each person is unique and needs to do things in his or her own way.

This is the time to give full acceptance, support, and comfort to the dying patient. Approximately one to three months prior to death, food and fluid intake will start to decrease, one may see an increase in confusion, increase in sleep, decrease in strength in legs and arms, withdrawal from the world and people, and bowels and bladder may become incontinent. Several weeks prior to death, the person's voice may become weaker, there may be more difficulty swallowing (dysphasia), restlessness, change in breathing patterns may be noticed (called Cheyne-Stokes), which is an oscillation of breathing from faster to slower with a period of apnea. Possibly seeing and talking to the deceased and a decrease in urinary output will be noticed as well. Days to hours prior to death, gurgling sounds are common (some refer to this as the death rattle). Other symptoms are an inability to swallow, no urine output, relaxed in the earlobe or the entire ear, relaxed lower jaw, restlessness or no activity at all, a surge of energy followed by no activity, fever, unable to close eyelids, hyperextended neck, increased change in breathing patterns. Minutes away from death, the patient becomes comatose and "fish out of water" breathing. So how do you recognize when death has occurred? No breathing or heartbeat, release of bowel and bladder, no response, eyelids slightly open, pupils enlarged, eyes fixed on a certain spot, no blinking, jaw relaxed with mouth slightly open. *(Durham, Weiss, 1997 & Karnes, 2009)*

So now that we went through the breakdown, let's explore a little deeper what this all means and what you can do as a caregiver.

The following signs and symptoms described are indicative of how the body physically prepares itself for the final stages of life.

Coolness: The person's hands, arms, and feet may be increasingly cool to the touch, and at the same time the color of the skin may change. This is a normal indication that the circulation of blood is decreasing to the body's extremities and being reserved for the most vital organs. Keep the person warm with a blanket, not an electric blanket. Speak softly, naturally, and directly to the patient as you normally would, even though there may be no response, and never assume that the person cannot hear you, as hearing is the last of the senses to be lost.

Disorientation: The person may seem to be confused about the time, place, and identity of people surrounding him or her, including close and familiar people. This is due, in part, to metabolism changes. Identify yourself by name before you speak rather than ask the person to guess who you are. Speak softly, clearly, and truthfully when you need to communicate something important for the patient's comfort, such as "it is time to take your medication." Then explain the reason for the communication, such as, "So you won't begin to hurt."

Incontinence: The person may lose control of urine and bowels as the muscles in that area begin to relax. This can be embarrassing to the patient and the family, so treat this with as much dignity as possible. Along with incontinence, the urine may decrease. This is a normal process. Urine also may become tea-colored due to its concentration. This is due to the decrease in fluid intake as well as a decrease in circulation through the kidneys. Sometimes inserting a catheter won't bring much of a result and may do more harm than good.

Congestion: The person may have gurgling sounds coming from his or her chest as though marbles are rolling around inside, and these sounds may become very loud. This is a normal change due to the decrease of fluid intake and an inability to cough up normal secretions. Suctioning usually only increases the secretions and can cause sharp discomfort. Gently turn the person's head to the side and allow gravity to drain the secretions. You may also gently wipe the mouth with a moist cloth. The sound of the congestion does not indicate the onset of severe or new pain.

Restlessness: The patient may make restless and repetitive motions, such as pulling at the bed linen or clothing. This often happens and is due, in part, to the decrease in oxygen circulation to the brain and to metabolism changes. Do not interfere with or try to restrain such motions. To have a calming effect, speak in a quiet, natural way, lightly massage the forehead, read to the person, or play some soothing music.

Decrease in food and fluid: The person will have a decrease in appetite and thirst, wanting little or no food or fluid. The body will naturally begin to conserve energy, which is expended on these tasks. Do not try to force food or fluid into the person or try to use guilt or manipulate them into eating or drinking something. Taste buds change as you get older, and things that people used to love, they may not like anymore. Small chips of ice, frozen Gatorade, popsicles, or juice may be given. If the person is able to swallow, fluid may be given in small amounts by syringe. If this is done, be trained first so the patient doesn't aspirate. Glycerin swabs may help keep the mouth and lips moist and comfortable. A cool, moist washcloth on the forehead may also increase physical comfort.

The following signs and symptoms are indicative of how the patient prepares emotionally, spiritually, and mentally for the final stage of life. This is a general guideline, compiled over the years by working with dying patients. Remember again that not everyone will go through these. However, the more you know, the more you will understand when that person does display these signs.

Withdrawal: The person may seem unresponsive, withdrawn, or in a comatose-like state. This indicates preparation for release, detaching from surroundings and relationships, and a beginning of letting go. Hearing remains all the way to the end, so speak to the person in your normal tone of voice, identifying yourself by name when you speak, hold his or her hand and say whatever you need to say that will help that person let go.

Vision-like experiences: The patient may speak to or claim to have spoken to persons who have already died, or to see or have seen places not presently accessible or visible to you. This does not indicate a drug reaction or a hallucination.

The patient is beginning to detach from this life and is being prepared for the transition so it will not be frightening for that person, although it may be scary to the family. Do not contradict, explain away, belittle, or argue about what the person claims to have seen or heard. Affirm the person's experience. These experiences are normal and common.

Decreased socialization: The person may only want to be with a very few or even just one person. This is a sign of preparation for release and affirms from whom the support is most needed in order to make the appropriate transition. If a loved one is not part of the inner circle at the end of life, it does not mean that they are not loved or are unimportant. It means that they have fulfilled their task with the person and it is time for them to say goodbye. As part of the inner circle, the loved one needs to affirm and support and give their permission to the dying person.

Unusual communication: The person may make a seemingly out-of-character on non sequitur statement, gesture, or request. This indicates that he or she is ready to say goodbye and is testing their loved ones to see if they are ready to let him or her go. These moments should be accepted as beautiful gifts when offered.

Giving permission: Giving permission by a loved one to let go without making the person feel guilty for leaving can be difficult. A dying person will normally try to hold on, even though it brings prolonged discomfort, in order to be sure those who are going to be left behind will be all right. The ability to release the dying person from this concern and give them assurance that it is all right to let go whenever he or she is ready is one of the greatest gifts one can give their loved one.

Saying goodbye: When the person is ready to die and the loved one is able to let go, then it is time to say goodbye. Saying goodbye is your final gift of love to the person. It allows the person closure and makes the final release possible. Tears are a normal and natural part of saying goodbye. Tears do not need to be hidden from the person or apologized for. Tears express love and help to let go.

Understanding the final message of the dying: Frequently, people who are dying will say things that seem hallucinatory. Jumbled and rambling as they may be, these final communications often hold important meaning for those who are leaving this world and for those whom they're leaving behind. If we listen carefully and gently, we may be able to understand what the dying are struggling to say. Sometimes they're telling us what's happening to them in those last hours or weeks. Sometimes they're asking for something that will help them die peacefully. By helping to interpret these hidden messages, we can ease the anxiety of patients and family members and help them find a special closeness.

In summary:

Recurring themes of the dying: 1) Being in the presence of the dead. The dying often talk to or "see" someone who has died.

2) Preparing to travel. Dying people often talk of going on a trip, packing their bags to begin their journey. 3) Seeing a place. Many dying people have a glimpse of "another world." Others speak of having a "dream" or a feeling of being in another place." This can occur weeks before the time of death or when death is imminent. 4) Choosing when to die. It is not uncommon for the dying to seem to cling to life until a loved one arrives. They also wait until a loved one leaves before dying. 5) Knowing the time of death. Many times, the message the dying give is that they are about to die. They may say goodbye to their loved ones indirectly or directly.

So how do you respond to the dying? Respond in ways that tell them you accept whatever they say or see. Follow up what they say in a gentle way. Ask questions and offer sensitively probing insights that might encourage them to keep talking. Ask them to repeat statements if you don't understand what they are trying to say. For example, you might say, I am not sure I follow what you are telling me. Can you explain that a little more? Accept them regardless of how they appear to be responding to the impending death. For example, if they're having difficulty letting go, don't deny the problem; acknowledge it and offer help. Don't push the patient to talk. If they don't want to visit with you, then drop it; they have to be ready. At the same time, reinforce that you're still interested whenever they want to talk.

There are certain things that one can do to soften the mood and relax the patient. Aromatherapy is a proven method of relaxing someone. Think back to some of the pleasant aromas that you have smelt over the years. Use aromas the patient used to like and add them to the room. Play soft music of what the patient used to listen to. Pet therapy is a great way to relax someone; bring in their dog, cat, or whatever they had and let that animal lay in the bed with the person. This can bring on great relief and release in a person. A gentle massage, Reiki therapy, whatever the person was into before that will help them relax, then do if appropriate at that time. This brings on a sense of comfort and relaxation in the person and may help them release the energy that needs to be released to pass on.

Chapter 3

Psychology: Attitudes of Aging, Death, and Dying

The psychological process of dying is a complex area to cover. The experience of dying varies with age. The elderly think and talk about dying and are less afraid of death than the younger generations, and of course this varies with life experiences, personalities, religious beliefs, and their personal acceptance of death and dying. In years of working with clients (families and patients), the ones who struggle the most are the families, and of course they are the ones that are being left behind. The patients, for the most part, accept the inevitable.

Let's look at this from an elder point of view. As the baby boomers enter the retirement years, their social contacts or network of friends start to diminish. The colleagues they worked with move away or die off. Their kids are grown and have their own kids and lives. Elderly people not wanting to be a burden keep more to themselves, don't disclose to their kids what they are going through or how they are feeling; they just fade off into the sunset.

If you have taken any courses in human relations or psychology, one name that has probably been brought up is Abraham Maslow's (1908-1970) hierarchy of needs *(Kleinman, 2012)*, and as he states, these needs are basic for survival. All others are secondary. These hierarchies of needs are in a pyramid shape, and according to Maslow's law, the lower-level needs must be satisfied before moving up the pyramid to the next level.

The first need, which is the bottom part of the pyramid, is physiological. These are the basic needs: food, water, air, and sleep. Just as newborns and infants depend only on these needs, the elderly as they get older fall back to these basic needs. Their intake decreases, which decreases their strength, and which affects their bodily functions, heart, kidneys, brain, etc. When this happens, the body goes into a homeostasis imbalance, which causes disease and eventually death. This is a big area that families and caregivers tend to neglect, the basic needs. Over the years, patients have told me that they are hungry, thirsty, need to be cleaned, and so how can caregivers ignore these basic needs?

This is a two-part question/answer. The elderly tend to sleep more often than the younger population, and so they don't get the food/fluid that they need during the day. The other reason is that the caregivers are not educated as to the nutritional needs of the elderly. They tend to feel that two to three meals a day are sufficient. This is not the case. The elderly person tends to eat less of each meal, which requires smaller, more frequent meals during the day. For instance, if for lunch a person only eats half a sandwich and has a little water and says they are done, then the caregiver may assume that they don't need anything else until dinner. Keeping nutritious snacks available will help that person meet their nutritional needs. Also, the elderly don't want to be a bother for their kids or caregivers, so they won't ask for anything else to eat or drink. Remember, we all need nutrition to survive, and in the elderly and those with life-limiting illnesses, this is an important area not to neglect.

The second need is safety and security. As with infants, these are important to the geriatric population. This shows up as a safe place to live, caregivers that are honest and caring and that won't take advantage of their money or possessions. In my years of taking care of geriatric and critically ill patients, there was more and more abuse: physical, emotional, financial, and sexual. The economy plays a big role in this. When the economy declines, some of the elderly may have to live with adult children or vice versa. When an elderly person moves in with his or her children, this causes stress on that family, especially if that family has children of their own that the parents are taking care of. This stress may not only be physical but may be financial as well. If the adult child is financially strapped, he or she may use the parent's Social Security money to help them survive.

The abuse escalates when that child or caregiver holds back necessary medical services, medications, etc., to take care of their own needs, or when that elderly person is left alone all day, and their basic needs for elimination, food, and water are not being considered.

Verbal and physical abuse can arise out of frustration and stress, as the living quarters may be small, and the needs of that elderly person are overwhelming to the family. In the US, this is becoming a big problem as the baby boomers are reaching that age of retirement and are having more health issues. Their kids have to deal with trying to meet their needs along with their family's needs and work obligations. If there are a number of brothers and sisters in the picture, this can arise as arguments in the family unit as to how to take care of the parents, causing family fights, and possibly severing relationships.

In other countries, it is expected that the elderly will live with one of the children, and the other children will help in the care of their parents. As the world becomes more global, children moving away from their neighborhoods for college or career, we will see more issues in regard to taking care of our elderly. Remember, one day you too may be in this situation.

The third need in this pyramid is love and belonging. As with infants and children who want to feel love and that they belong, in the elderly population their social circle dwindles down to the point of maybe them having a couple of friends that they may talk to. You may notice this in your grandparent(s) or even parents. They become more and more dependent for this need with their families. They get very lonely, and when this elderly person gets to be more homebound, this loneliness escalates. Their kids are at work, their friends are few, and they may be too crippled to leave home without being assisted. For the families, they become more and more burdensome. This brings stress on to the family and may affect this love and belonging feeling in the elderly. You can see the cyclic effect here. Remember how children are dependent at birth and their early years of growing; most of the elderly are the same; they want to be accepted and feel loved like when they were younger. As my grandmother expressed to my mom, who told me what she said. My grandmother living alone said, "I'm as lonely as a dog."

This ties into the fourth layer on this pyramid, which is self-esteem. This is a huge issue in the elderly population, especially in the very old, where there is a loss of bowel functions (incontinence) and swallowing problems (dysphasia). If the elder person is alert and orientated, this can very humiliating. In a baby, the incontinence, drooling, and frequent spitting up is normal. The infant doesn't know any better. However, the elderly person does, if they have their faculties. Imagine for a moment you are dependent on someone, having to clean you up after a bowel movement, having to feed and clean you, bathe you. This loss of self-esteem is hard psychologically. They now are dependent on someone else and feel the loss of respect they once had and the humiliation that goes along with loss of privacy. In residential homes (group homes), assisted living facilities, or nursing homes where the elderly go to for their needs to be met, they feel this loss of self-esteem on a daily basis. They not only depend on their physical needs to be met, but their social needs as well. Some facilities are very well established in meeting these needs with social activities, but more importantly, the dignity of the person is respected. When this is accomplished, the elderly person feels respected by others, and this gives them a feeling of joy and love that they so much desire.

The top of the pyramid is self-actualization. The elderly may or may not reach this level in their lifetime. In the elderly, they do reflect on their life, the accomplishments they made, the mistakes, the things that they have done or wish they had done; all this comes into play. They are at a point that they can't reach whatever goal they wanted, which may cause distress, depression, anger, or they may feel satisfied with the goals they accomplished. They are happy and not concerned with the ones they didn't accomplish. This is their self-actualization.

Five stages of grief:

Let's focus now on Dr. Elisabeth Kubler-Ross's five stages of grief. *(Kubler-Ross, 1969)* Almost everyone has heard of Dr. Elisabeth Kubler-Ross and her five stages of grief and what a patient goes through from first finding out that their life has an end point. These stages are quite important, although I need to point out that people go through their grief in different ways and in different time phases. These stages are guidelines, not set in stone to follow; however, it is important to look at these stages and what a person may go through, these are:

1. Denial and isolation (no, not me): This is a survival mechanism of the conscious ego, which helps the unconscious mind to evaluate the situation. The other saying in psychology

is the fight/flight response. When people get bad news about their health, and once the shock has worn off, that person, with encouragement and advice by the family, will usually seek out other medical opinions, other treatments, faith healers, shamans (fight response), or will go into complete isolation, shunning family, friends, or anyone wanting to help them (flight). Humans are encoded with this fight/flight mechanism, so they will do and pay for what sounds the best for them to beat this disease and live. This person may want blood transfusions, medical tests, and surgery, even though the doctors say that it won't help. Actually, what it comes down to is that people want hope and a lot of time false assurances that they will beat this and live to a ripe old age.

2. Anger (Why me?): Once the denial phase has faded away or can't be maintained, it is replaced with feelings of anger, resentment, and ridicule directed to staff, family, friends, or anyone in reach of their wrath. Anger may be small and specific, such as the lab having to redo a test, to very large and philosophical, such as God, why did you let this happen to me? They will often say, why is this happening to me? I don't deserve this. What about that eighty-year-old lady that is happy, living independently, goes to play bingo every night, and I am stuck in this room, this bed, or whatever the case may be. This person may say, I have been good, I worked hard all my life, and I don't deserve this. This person may have wished they had taken that Italy trip sooner or learned to play that piano that is sitting in the corner, but they had been too busy. All these reactions come into play in the anger phase, which is hard for family and friends to deal with. They may feel that the anger is directly targeted at them; they may feel helpless, scared, and unsure of what to do for that person. The family reaction is to respond with sadness, tears, decreasing visits, even responding with their own anger.

3. Bargaining or guilt: When denial and anger don't seem to be working, then the person will usually resort to bargaining. If you have children, you know about this stage. If they ask for something and you say no, initially they will get angry, maybe throw a tantrum, and stomp off to their room. Once that is over, they will start to think of other ways to get what they want; this is usually bargaining. "I will wash the car, clothes, dishes for a week if you let me do this, have that."

This is no different in people that have a life-limiting illness or disease. They will ask God, if you can let me do this one thing, take this trip, or whatever it is, then I will accept this disease and suffering. No one really thinks about dying. We are all wrapped up in our own lives until something happens and we hit a brick wall that stops us in our tracks, and we then realize, oh no, now what? This bargaining is a psychological process we all do. Guilt plays a big role in this, and people will feel that if they had treated others better, given more to charities, worked at homeless shelters, then they might have been spared this dreaded illness or disease. We all do it, whether consciously or not.

4. Depression: This is the stage (after the fighting, bargaining, denying, endless treatments, tests, surgeries) where the person starts to realize that this could be the end. This person now realizes that they may not be around to see their daughters or sons married, not able to dance at their weddings, or see their grandchildren grow and share in their lives. This person may also feel that he is not a man if he has testicular cancer and his testicles and penis have been removed, or a woman who had breast cancer and one or both of her breasts have been removed. This person realizes that a lot of money has been spent on finding a cure, but there was none. Now their savings are depleted, they may have lost their job, they may have to sell their house, all these play a role in this stage of depression. Elderly people are very

susceptible to this. As they get older and more frail, there will come a time when they can no longer live in their house where they lived for forty or fifty years and raised their family. Their children are becoming caretakers, burdened with their parent(s) and trying to raise their own family. It will be the children who decide that mom or dad needs to be in an environment where they can be monitored so to take the burden and the guilt off of them. The elderly realize that and do get very depressed when they are forced to leave their home. They end up in a group home, assisted living facility, or nursing home, depending on the severity of their illness. All their lives they worked hard and cared for their family, only to be "put out to pasture" as one gentleman told me. This can be especially hard on a person that was a socialite or very active in their community to now have to live a lonely life in a strange place without their friends, having very few visitors coming, family maybe coming once a week to see them and endless days of sitting in front of a TV or in a room with only a radio going with very little social activity.

Depression in the elderly is a big business for the pharmaceutical industry. Depression medication is prescribed like candy to the elderly because family tell the doctor that mom/dad seems depressed, sad, crying a lot, so the physician will prescribe an antidepressant for them. Whereas what the family needs to do is ask them why they are sad or depressed, and usually they will tell them. Giving medication is more of a convenience for the family to keep their parents happy, and this helps the caregiver's guilt.

So, let's get to the root of things. Depression is a way for a person to start to realize their loss, loss of freedom, financial independence, friends, family, and the realization of impending death. Nothing is worse than to lose friends that one had for many years or to have family in other states where they only visit a couple times a year. Loss is hard on a person, especially the elderly. They start to feel that they are a burden on society or their families, and so their depression spirals down to where sometimes they revert back to their childhood or go within themselves, holding their blanket, pillow, or doll. They babble, drool, and become incontinent, where they weren't like this before, and now more pills are given until the person becomes a zombie.

5. Acceptance: This is the stage where the person accepts their fate. They have come to terms with the time they have left. They may become emotionally detached from their illness and maybe the world. They will start to enjoy the little things in life, like sitting outside and listening, really listening to the bird's chirp. They have a new appreciation of how flowers smell in the spring or the feel of a summer breeze. They don't really care about the world around them. Their focus is on enjoying family and friends. They remove the nonessential clutter of life and focus on the essentials of relationships. One may see a total personality change in the person. Maybe they were standoffish, grumpy, or an introvert; now they are open, talking, and smiling all the time, wanting to be involved with their grandchildren more. At first, this could throw off people that know this person, expressing wonderment at the changes they see.

So how does one encourage and support this person as they go through their journey? There are a number of ways to do this. One is reflective listening, developed by Carl Rogers, focused on the client-centered therapy in counseling theory. *(Kleinman, 2012)*

In this client-centered therapy, Rogers believed that a client was ultimately in charge of their happiness. The use of reflective listening is a communication strategy involving two key steps: Seeking to understand a speaker's idea, in this case the elderly person, then offering the idea back to the speaker to confirm the idea has been understood correctly. It attempts to reconstruct what the person is thinking and feeling and to relay this understanding back to the person, one then actively engages in the conversation by reducing or eliminating distractions of any kind to allow for paying full attention to the conversation at hand. *(Lane, 2005)*

In other words, really listen to what the person is telling you. They are struggling with their life issues, and they really want someone to listen to them. In their view this may be the last time they talk or see you, and they so desperately want to share their fears, stories, or whatever it may be with you. So let them talk. This can be the greatest gift you can give to that person before they die, the gift of caring.

Chapter 4

Right to Die

Euthanasia, assisted suicide, mercy killing, these areas are all lumped into this chapter because they are all intertwined; they all have different names but mean essentially the same thing. Assisted suicide is where the person takes his or her own life with the assistance of someone else, especially a physician, and euthanasia is where a doctor ends the patient's life. This area is a growing concern among people dealing with their own life-limiting illness or with a family member that has a life-limiting illness. Laws are in place to forbid assisted suicides, mercy killings, etc., but a number of states are starting to legalize this. So, what does this mean? Euthanasia, physician-assisted suicide, mercy killing is a practice of intentionally ending a life in order to relieve pain and suffering. The right to die relates to or advocates a person's right to refuse measures intended to prolong life after a physician has deemed that person to be terminally ill. *(The American Heritage Medical Dictionary, 2008)*

Let's explore this more closely. As we age, our body slows down, eyesight fails, cognitive skills decline, we have more aches and pains than when we did when we were younger, our organs slow down, taste buds change, intake of food and fluids lessen, dehydration becomes more of a problem, along with urinary tract infections. For most people, they have more pain, and relieving this pain is a challenge for medical personnel. There is a delicate balance between relieving pain and overdosing someone on painkillers. People with cancer usually experience a lot of pain, depending on where the cancer is. For the thousands who go through this pain, if not managed correctly, this can lead them to think about suicide. Normally in the beginning of a cancer diagnosis, or for that matter any diagnosis of a life-ending disease, the patient will usually go through the treatments, hoping for a cure. Younger patients will fight and use every means to look for a cure to this disease. Whereas an older person, also hoping for a cure, is more realistic and will go through the treatments, however they may cut the treatments short, knowing the treatments are causing more pain and discomfort and are not working, then all they want is to be out of pain and comfortable until the end.

The goal of the medical community is to alleviate pain and keep the patient as comfortable as possible, and to achieve this different medications are given. Sometimes, though, this brings on a death that is quicker than the family expects, leaving guilt and questions as if the medication caused the death. There is a term used in the medical community called double effect. The doctrine or principle of double effect is often invoked to explain the permissibility of an action that causes serious harm, such as the death of a human being, as a side effect of promoting some good end. It is claimed that sometimes it is permissible to cause such harm as a side effect (or double effect) of bringing about a good result. The double effect means sometimes it is permissible to bring about a harmful event that otherwise would be impermissible to bring about intentionally. *(Stanford Encyclopedia of Philosophy, 2013)*

For example, giving a person morphine is intended to relieve pain. However, if this person has low blood pressure and is semi-comatose, the unintended effect can be death. Another example is when a person loses the ability to swallow, and family or that person refuses an alternative way of nutrition, which is a feeding tube, or asks to withdraw this feeding, then without that nutrition that person will eventually die.

One must remember if the person is alert and orientated to self and others and is of sound mind and chooses to not take medication or refuses artificial feedings or just refuses to eat, then there is not much one can do; that is their choice. Let's make this point clear, when an adult chooses—the operative word here is chooses—not to care for himself or herself in any way to treat their condition, that is their choice. Courts will usually overrule people trying to control a person that has their mental capacities and chooses their own fate. If a person is a minor, that is a different story; the courts will either choose a guardian or appoint someone to make those decisions if the parents are out of the picture.

Choosing suicide, euthanasia, and mercy killing is against the law, unless the state legalizes it. Federal law trumps state law, as in the case of marijuana. Usually the federal government will stay away from the issues of suicide, euthanasia, and mercy killing as long as it is legal in that state and handled correctly.

The question arises, why keep people alive when we know their time is near? For one thing, when people are on chemotherapy, physicians (remember their Hippocratic oath) want to keep the patient going, even though they know what the outcome is because it is their duty to do everything in their power to keep that patient alive. Other reasons include families' and patients' beliefs, cultural upbringing, hopes for a cure to come through, and denial that the person is dying. In the course of my practice I have seen many families send their loved ones to the hospital when clearly the patient is dying; they want that one last shot of keeping them alive. When the family is living off the Social Security of the patient, of course they want that person to live as long as possible. Group homes or residential homes depend on this revenue since this person living there represents their revenue, and once that patient dies, so does their revenue.

When people have too much pain and nothing is working, they want to end their suffering. This is where different societies have popped up, like the Hemlock Society, founded in 1980. Its mission is to educate people who want to hasten their death due to debilitating diseases and to push legislation for physician-assisted suicide. In 2003, the nonprofit society changed its name and merged to be called Compassion and Choices. Over the years, states have tried and most failed to get legislation passed on physician-assisted suicide.

There are four states at this time that allow physician-assisted suicide; these are Oregon, Washington, Montana, and Vermont. Oregon and Washington passed their laws by public vote. Vermont enacted the law legislatively, and Montana's supreme court ruled that physicians may aid terminally ill patients in dying if they requested it. *(Hallenbeck, 2013)* So the process is set forth in law, including the requirements that the patient must be of sound mind when requesting assisted suicide, as confirmed by a doctor and other witnesses, and the patient must be diagnosed with a terminal illness. There are other states at this time working on legislation for this, however, no other states have passed this law.

There was one doctor who brought this issue out in the open in the 1990s, and he was Dr. Jack Kevorkian, who assisted over one hundred people in Michigan to commit suicide due to a debilitating disease. Since there were no laws set up, he was never charged. The last person he helped, he actually assisted in killing the patient and aired it on *60 Minutes*. He was found guilty and served eight years. He was released in 2007 and died in 2011. Dr. Kevorkian believed that people had a right to die if they so choose due to a debilitating disease; unfortunately, he crossed that proverbial line. His actions have pushed this issue to the forefront of people's minds as to the legal and ethical issues.

As people develop incurable cancers or debilitating diseases like ALS or multiple sclerosis, as the disease progresses people become bedridden, are in pain, and develop bedsores. They are totally dependent on someone to care for them 24–7. Most people don't want to live like this. There was a woman in her forties that had advanced multiple sclerosis. She was living in a nursing home, and one day she decided enough was enough and stopped eating. Legally, there was nothing the nurses, doctor, the facility, or the family could do, as this patient was alert and orientated to self and others and had made that choice for herself, and she eventually died. Another lady had end-stage ALS. She was bedridden, and the only way she could communicate was with a light on her head, pointing it to a letter board and spelling out the words. Her wish was not to go on a ventilator with a feeding tube. At the point of her disease worsening, she was given a morphine drip, which sedated her, keeping her comfortable, and eventually she died. Now you say that is physician-assisted suicide, right? Actually, this is what is called palliative sedation. This patient was aware, and it was her choice to choose this method. Here is the double effect scenario; morphine was given to keep her comfortable, and the end effect was her death.

Palliative sedation:

Palliative sedation is the practice of relieving distress in a terminally ill person in their last days or hours of life by using an infusion of a sedative drug. This option is for people whose symptoms cannot be controlled by any other means. The goal is to control symptoms of a patient through sedation until the person dies, as opposed to euthanasia or physician-assisted suicide, where it shortens the patient's life to cease suffering. Again, this is a fine line, as one can argue that without this sedation the patient would have lived longer, days or maybe weeks. The *Journal of the American Medical Association (JAMA)* states it this way. Palliative sedation is the use of sedative medications to relieve extreme suffering by making the patient unaware and unconscious (as in a deep sleep) while the disease takes its course, eventually leading to death. The sedative medication is gradually increased until the patient is comfortable and able to relax. Palliative sedation is not intended to cause death or shorten life. *(JAMA, 2005)* So in our example of the lady that had ALS, she was given palliative sedation so she wouldn't suffer the feeling of asphyxiation. The last muscles to go in ALS are the respiratory muscles, and if you ever had asthma or bronchitis, you know how scary the feeling is when you can't breathe. In her case, palliative sedation was justified and was her choice.

Palliative care is different than palliative sedation. Palliative care is comfort care, so when a patient decides enough is enough, no more chemo, no more tests, no more surgeries, etc., and that they just want to be comfortable and out of pain, this is when palliative care takes over. JAMA defines it thusly: Palliative care provides comfort care to the patient by focusing on relieving symptoms such as pain, anxiety, nausea, and difficulty breathing. Family members as well as the patient are provided with emotional, social, and spiritual support to help them with the dying process. *(JAMA, 2005)*

For a person to be comfortable, certain medications may be given in lieu of treatments. For most physicians, they defer this type of care to physicians and organizations that deal with this specialty of healthcare, and these organizations are called hospices. Let's talk about hospice and what it is and what it does. First, let's look at the history of hospice and how it started. Hospice comes from the Latin term hospitium, which means hospitality. In olden days, knights hospitallers evolved in response to the Crusades, where people cared for the knights that fought in the Crusades, and over the course of time this is how hospitals evolved. In 1965, Dame Cicely Saunders, a nurse and social worker and who eventually became a physician, recognized the need for people to die with dignity and pain-free. She founded St. Christopher hospice in England in 1967 and traveled to the US to spread the word. The first US hospice was started in New Haven, Connecticut, and began services in 1974.

What is the hospice philosophy? It refers to a concept of compassionate care for people in the final phases of an incurable illness. It is to give the family and patient sensitivity and support and to treat people with respect and dignity. Hospice seeks neither to hasten nor postpone death. The emphasis is on quality of life and dignity. Next is symptom management, which is the key to the quality of life of a patient near the end. This care is always guided by a team, which includes a medical director, nurse, social worker, chaplain, home health aide, and volunteers in collaboration with the family and patient. This also includes, after the patient dies, bereavement support for the family, which lasts for thirteen months and includes the anniversary of the patient's death. Some facts and figures: hospices have been growing steadily since 1974, where there was one. By 2009 there was over 5,000, and the number is still climbing today. In 2011 an estimated 1.65 million patients received services under hospice care, which represents 44.6 percent of deaths. *(NHPCO, 2012)* As you can see, hospice services are rising each year as the baby boomers become older and are appropriate for hospice care. To be eligible for hospice care, the physician has to certify that based on the disease process, the patient has less than six months to live. This is not concrete, as patients can live from one month to a year after their diagnosis. This is a physician's best guess based on the patient's disease and all the documentation that the doctor has. There is one interesting fact. In a press release in 2011 by the NHPCO, it states that there was a drop in the length of stay for hospice patients in 2009, meaning that they came on later and died sooner. In their report they state that hospice providers are not reaching the patients sooner. Also, in previous decades, hospices overwhelmingly cared for people with cancer. In 2010, cancer diagnoses dropped to 35.6 percent from 40 percent in 2009. Now heart disease is the leading diagnosis under hospice. *(NHPCO, 2012)* As was mentioned, as medical technology and treatments grow, so does the hope of people to live longer, using all means to get treated, and when this doesn't work and death is approaching, most go on hospice and die fairly soon after being admitted, while some fight until the end, never going onto hospice care.

If hospices are in place for relieving pain and symptom management, then why euthanasia or physician-assisted suicide? Pain and symptom management is the goal for hospices. But the bottom line is that people living with pain and a crippling disease like ALS or MS don't want to live like that, and the hospice philosophy does not support ending life. People look for alternatives, as in euthanasia or physician-assisted suicide, and the right to die will be a hot topic for years to come.

Chapter 5

Grief & Spirituality

Grief is the intense emotional response to the pain of a loss. It is the reflection of a connection that has been broken. Most important, grief is an emotional, spiritual, and psychological journey to healing. *(Kubler-Ross & Kessler, 2005)*

Mourning is the psychological process that occurs when you experience loss. *(Cooper & McKesson, 2001)*

Watching a loved one die or experiencing a death is hard for anyone, even for the experienced person. People experience death in their own way and their own time. Some internalize death; others display their emotions very outwardly. Again, let's look at Elisabeth Kubler-Ross's stages: denial, anger, guilt, bargaining, depression, and acceptance. These stages are experienced by the person that has a life-limiting illness, but what about the people that are left behind? They too, according to Dr. Kubler-Ross, go through these stages. These stages were developed to illuminate the life and dying process, where one has a terminal disease, and loved ones travel this journey along with the dying person. However, one must remember that these stages are fluid, not concrete. If someone is going through the grief process feels that they are not leaving one of these stages, then there must be something wrong. Remember, there are different types of grief. They range from the grief that your son or daughter is going away to college, loss of a prized possession, death of a pet, having to move away from the neighborhood you grew up in, reestablishing yourself and your family to a new neighborhood, new school, new job, new life, grief over a divorce, having to start over again. If someone dies unexpectedly by heart attack, drowning, murder, suicide, or in the death of an infant or child, then the grief process is different and harder because the survivors were not expecting it. Survivors will flow through these stages but may bounce back and forth between the different stages, which actually is a more normal reaction to grief.

Reconciling the loss of a close loved one generally requires several years. Usually in the first year the survivor has memories and experiences of reliving their life with that loved one, recounting their trips, moments, fights, laughter, etc. Their grief is deep and painful, which is emotional grief. Usually the hardest moments in this first year of the grief process are the holidays, birthdays, and special occasions that they may have shared together and the anniversary of that person's death. Once this first year is over, the second year the survivor is adjusting to being without their loved one. Thinking of the things that were done without that person, the survivor is now beginning to build experiences and a life without that person. Subsequent years bring greater detachment; the survivor moves on with their life, developing other relationships or friendships and building new experiences.

Not to say grief disappears altogether. Grief will be like a roller coaster; it will have its ups and downs, especially during the holidays. However, over time this wave will smooth out. We are all human, so we experience grief in many ways, and our emotions manifest themselves either in healthy or unhealthy grief.

Recovery vs. reconciliation:

People often get this confused. Reconciliation means that one accepts what has happened, and recovery means a return to a normal state of health, mind, or strength. A survivor does not recover from the loss but reconciles the loss, accepts it, and once that is understood, that survivor can move on.

There are a number of factors that influence the grief process of the survivor. There are the cultural and circumstantial factors. Was the death expected or not? Social, relationship, and psychological factors may play a factor in how people get through the grief process.

Cultural: As explained earlier, everyone is brought up in some kind of culture or ethnicity. The values of that culture can have a profound effect on the recovery of a person experiencing loss. How close was that person to the deceased? Is that person spiritual or religious? (Is there a heaven where my wife/husband/son/daughter may be, and are they happy now?) Are the survivors more materialistic or nonbelievers of an afterlife? Is the culture stoic or does it show outward emotion? How did the circumstantial factors relate to the timing of the death? Were the survivors ready for the death or was it a surprise? Did the survivors have time to put into place the necessary arrangements? Were they prepared for the death? When people are ready for the person to die, the mourning process seems to be smoother and the length of the grief seems to be less. This is because people were prepared.

Now, there are a number of cases that the survivors were aware but stayed in denial, stating Mom/Dad or whoever it is will beat this, and when the person does pass away, they are in a state of shock, surprised, refusing to believe that they died. This enhances and prolongs the grief process due to the fact that those people were in denial and didn't want to accept this. These are the people you will see lash out, be angry, blame everyone else, or blame the person that died because they didn't fight enough or gave up.

Was the death sudden and unexpected? Being in a global world, as kids move away and settle somewhere else, were they even aware of the pending death? How close was that person to the deceased? Not being a part of the process can put guilt on the survivor. How much stress is on that person's life, and did the death cause more stress? Are the social and relational factors surrounding the death of a loved one important? That is, how close was that person to the deceased. Was there a love/hate relationship between the two? Were their lives intertwined or distant, being just friends? Was there unfinished business between the survivor and the deceased, unresolved issues that will never be resolved now? Psychological issues can be devastating to the survivor. Were their lives codependent? Were there self-esteem issues, psychological issues with the survivor where they may not understand the impact of that person's death on them? Did the person that was dying give permission to that person to move on, to enjoy their life, or was that person selfish up to the end? How much control did that person have over the survivor? If the dying person controlled the survivor's life, the survivor could be at a loss to make decisions, as they really never had to before.

As you can see from the above, there are a lot of factors that play into the grief process of the survivors, and there is no one answer. There are many books and therapists out there that will impose or explain what they think you should do to deal with the situation. The only way one can deal with grief once death is experienced is one needs to deal with it in a way that is healthy for them.

Dr. William Worden developed four tasks of grief, these are: *(Worden's, 2008)*

Accepting the reality of the loss: Initially, denial is a coping mechanism that most people tend to use; however, it is not healthy in the long run. Viewing the body is a way of accepting the finality of the person's death.

Accepting that grief is painful: One needs to embrace that pain, explore it, and accept it in order to move on.

Adjusting to an environment that no longer includes the deceased: The survivors need to adjust to the tasks and responsibilities without that other person. They need to develop their own routines and to move on without that person.

Withdrawing emotionally from the energy once given and moving on with their life: Hanging on to the guilt of that person's death is not healthy physically or psychologically; one needs to move on and reinvest that energy into a healthier lifestyle.

Most people get through this tough time relying on family, friends, and faith. Faith for most people is comforting, saying that God decided it was their time, they are happy now, and they are at peace. So how does spirituality play in this roll of death, dying, and grief? First, one must understand spirituality vs. religion. There are a lot of definitions to spirituality and religion. To put this into a simple context, spirituality is the belief of the spirit world to transcend this earthly plane and go to a place or belief beyond this realm. The spiritual dimension permeates all of life and strives for answers about the infinite, and especially comes into focus as a sustaining power when the person faces emotional stress, illness, or death. *(Murray, Zentner, Yakimo. 2009)*

Whereas religion is a fundamental belief in a higher power and a set of beliefs and practices agreed upon by a set of people, for example, Catholic, Buddhists, Christian, Jewish, etc. Religion includes a belief in a supernatural or divine force that has power over the universe and commands worship and obedience to a supernatural force, a set of practices that are followed, and a church affiliation. *(Murray, Zentner, Yakimo. 2009)*

Everyone has their own view of an afterlife; some believe strongly in God or a supreme being, and others believe that once you die that is it. This is a touchy subject to write about. Only that person who is dying and those close to that person can justify in their minds what they want to believe in.

Grief includes a desire that people want it to be like before. Death really messes up one's plans, and it disrupts lives. People either get really angry with God, questioning their faith, or they go way overboard and pray constantly, asking God to forgive their sins as this must be why that person died. Grief has physical consequences; we have heartache, stomach pains, and depression so severe we may have to go on medication. Depression can be an issue for people not handling death well. If someone has a diagnosis of depression already or psychotic issues like bipolar or schizophrenia, this can become a bigger problem. Fear plays a big role in physical pain, as it can remind us of our mortality and how we have less control over our lives than we thought.

How do we work through this grief process? As mentioned above, some people rely on their faith and their families to get them through this time. Some medicate themselves, and some just bury the grief or guilt. When someone first dies, people are in a state of shock and numbness. They go through the motions of making arrangements for the funeral, burial, and cremation. They surround themselves with family and friends, but once that is all over, they realize they are alone. This is where their faith and spirituality may kick in. They realize they need something more to help them through this tough time.

Over time, this grieving process may wean down. In five or ten years, people may have moved on with their lives, not forgetting the person that passed on, but remembering the good times they had with them. What those people could do is acknowledge that loss, accept it for what it is, embrace it, and let it go, like letting go of doves at a wedding. No one can convey the depth of sadness they feel for their loss, but the strength of that person to work through it will create a new and fulfilling life.

As a hospice clergy once told me, what he does is have people write a grief letter. This letter describes what that person has experienced and how they are feeling about the loss or impending loss. For those people that are dying, they too can write a grief letter describing what they are feeling and then give a copy of this letter to their friends and family. This way, they know how that person that is dying feels, and this may help family and friends understand better what is going on and may ease the tension in the room.

Chapter 6

Ethics in Healthcare

In the previous chapters we discussed cultural and psychological issues, physiology of the dying process, grief and spirituality, and right to die. In all these chapters there is something that is in common with all this information, and that is ethical issues. For example, in your cultural beliefs, do you let Mom, Dad, Grandpa, or Grandma pass on if you believe that there may be a cure and you feel that they should keep fighting, and they say that they just want to be comfortable and die? Do you let someone decide to stop the feeding tube, even though you know it will cause his or her death? Your family member is in terrible pain, and your religion dictates that they are not to take any medications for this; however, this will help relieve their pain. Tough questions and tough decisions, aren't they? This is what ethics is all about—making tough choices, even though they may go against your beliefs or cultural ideology.

Ethics is about should and could, right from wrong; there is a fine line between ethics and legality. For example, if you see an accident happen in front of you and you see that everyone is okay and you are late for an appointment, do you stop or continue on? The law states that if you witness an accident, you are legally bound to stop and at least call for help. However, what if you are running late and don't have time to stop? Well, you could be cited for not stopping at an accident, however you made that important appointment, so that act may not be unethical.

What is ethics?

Ethics is a standard of behavior, developed as a result of one's concept of right and wrong.

A code of ethics is a guide for an individual or group to follow in making decisions regarding ethical issues.

What is ethics then? Ethics is not about religion, not about the society you live in, and not about the everyday things we do. What it is about is moral judgment, deciding from right and wrong. It is the conscious intent to do what is right, the conscious and deliberate effort in guiding one's conduct by reason based on fairness. *(Singer, 2011)* It is about choices, which are hard and can be tragic, because they can be about life and death, and the choices that are made by human beings. There are convincing arguments on both sides of an issue. There are no easy answers, no right or wrong; everything in an ethical decision is gray.

Let's look at a couple of scenarios:

You are a power of attorney (POA) for a family member. You are at the hospital and the doctor tells you that your loved one is comatose and the only way to keep them alive is to keep them on a ventilator and put in a feeding tube in the hope that he/she will wake up, or do you stop everything now and let them pass on? Let's say that your siblings are arguing both sides of this to influence your decision.

You are a nurse and the manager of a floor in a hospital or nursing home. You have a coworker that you have been best friends with since grade school that is working the floor. You both are working the evening shift, and you happen to be on the floor as your friend is passing medication. You see them take some narcotics that were intended for a patient and put them in their pocket. Remember, you two have been friends for a long time.

Easy for the reader to say, well, I would let them pass on, or I would report the nurse. From the outside looking in, decisions can be easy. But put yourself in their place, not so easy, is it? Here are other ethical dilemmas that healthcare workers may face: Prolonging someone's life in order for the family to see the patient before they die; withholding a blood transfusion from a baby whose parents are Jehovah witness; a patient continually asking you for antibiotics because they have a urinary tract infection or other infection; withholding information from a patient when a medication error was made, even though the outcome did not affect them in a negative manner.

Some definitions that are used in healthcare.

Autonomy comes from Latin, "auto," which means self, and "nomy," which means control. Individuals must be given the right to assist in their own decision-making. This ethical concept has led to the need for informed consent. In autonomy, patients' religious or cultural beliefs may lead them to make decisions regarding their own care that may seem controversial or even dangerous. However, the concept of autonomy gives them the right to make those decisions unless they are mentally impaired. *(Mosby, 2013 & Panza, Potthast, 2010)*

Beneficence means to do good, not harm, to other people. *(Mosby. 2013 & Panza, Potthast, 2010)*

Non-malfeasance is the concept of preventing intentional harm. Both of these ethical concepts relate directly to patient care. *(Mosby 2013 & Panza, Potthast, 2010)* In the American Nurses Association, Code for Nurses *(ANA. 1985)*, there is a specific charge to protect patients by specifying that nurses should report unsafe, illegal, or unethical practices by any person.

Nurses and physicians are often faced with making decisions about extending life with technology that might not be in the best interest of the patient. Often the concept of weighing potential benefit to the patient against potential harm is used in making these difficult decisions, along with the patient's own stated wishes.

Justice: The word justice is closely tied with the legal system. However, the word refers to the obligation to be fair to all people. Healthcare economics have hospitals and other providers stretching their resources to their limits. Economic decisions about healthcare resources have to be made based on the number of patients who would benefit. The potential of rationing care to the frail elderly, poor, and disabled creates an ethical dilemma that is sure to become even more complicated in the future.

Fidelity refers to the concept of keeping a commitment. Although the word is more closely used to describe a marital relationship, fidelity is the concept of accountability. What is the nurse/doctor's responsibility to his or her patient, employer, society, or government? Privacy and confidentiality are concepts that could be challenged under the concept of fidelity. If a nurse/doctor is aware of another healthcare giver who is impaired, but the circumstances are private or confidential, how is the conflict resolved?

Malfeasance is a comprehensive term used in both civil and criminal law to describe any act that is wrongful. It is not a distinct crime or tort but may be used generally to describe any act that is criminal or that is wrongful and gives rise to, or somehow contributes to, the injury of another person. *(Mosby, 2013 & Panza, Potthast, 2010)*

Let's take another scenario, which actually happened: A patient in a nursing home that you are taking care of has the later stages of multiple sclerosis, and she decides that she doesn't want to eat, drink, or take any medication—she said she just wants to die. She is alert and oriented to herself, place, and environment. In this case, because she was alert and orientated and had made her choice, there was not much one could do. The physician, social worker, chaplain, family, and I had talked with her, and this was brought up to an ethics committee, which I was a part of, and all agreed this was her choice and we honored her wishes. Eventually this patient did die, and as you can see this was an ethical dilemma that we in the healthcare field faced. We could not take this to court, as this patient was mentally fit, had signed all the proper documents, and made this her choice.

There is a term that was used in the euthanasia chapter called the *double effect*, again bringing this term to the ethics chapter. This doctrine or principle of double effect is giving a medication or doing something for one's good that however can cause harm, even death. These are the grey areas, the ethical choices that are made every day by families, health care professionals, and patients themselves. Their choice may result in their eventual death, as was the scenario of the patient that had MS. When giving a person enough morphine to control pain when the patient has low blood pressure, is semi-comatose, and is bedbound, the intent is to relieve pain and relax the respiratory system. However, in a person with these conditions, the unintended effect can be death.

Here is another example, a person loses the ability to swallow (dysphagia), and family or that person refuses an alternative way of nutrition (which is a feeding tube), or if that same patient has a feeding tube in place and is getting nutrition through this tube via a pump and then asks to withdraw the feeding. The end result is without that nutrition that person will eventually die. The ethical dilemma of the double effect is tricky. The nurse or doctor wants to keep the patient as comfortable as possible but knows that the possible outcome can be death.

The next step is to tell the family about the double effect, but how do you tell them? It is a known fact that in a crisis situation, such as when a family member is critically ill, the family and friends may hear only a fraction of what you're telling them and may only process part of that. If the patient does happen to pass on after receiving morphine for a few days, the family may question if the morphine (killed) the person, or too much was given that led to their death. Do you withhold some information in the beginning because of this?

The question is, is it ethical to withhold the truth from dying patients? Philosophers like Aristotle argued that truth is either an absolute value or at least preferable to deception. While others like Immanuel Kant, Henry Sidgwick, and others stated that deception might be acceptable in certain instances. If these and other philosophers cannot agree on this position, how can physicians be guided in their pursuit for truth and the desire to protect their patients from harm? The American Medical Association (AMA) code of ethics over the years has been amended to where it states in the 1980 AMA Principles of Medical Ethics that a physician shall deal honestly with patients and their colleagues. *(AMA code of medical ethics)*

In the American Hospital Association, The Patients' Bill of Rights was first adopted by the American Hospital Association in 1973 and revised in October 1992. Patient rights were developed with the expectation that hospitals and healthcare institutions would support these rights in the interest of delivering effective patient care. The American Hospital Association encourages institutions to translate or simplify the bill of rights to meet the needs of their specific patient populations and to make patient rights and responsibilities understandable to patients and their families. According to the American Hospital Association, a designated surrogate can exercise a patient's rights on their behalf if the patient lacks the decision-making capacity, is legally incompetent, or is a minor. *(AHA, 2002)*

The patient has the right to obtain from his or her physician complete and current information concerning their diagnosis, treatment, and prognosis in terms that the patient can reasonably expect to understand. Also, as a patient, you have certain rights, some of which are guaranteed by federal law, such as the right to get a copy of your medical records and the right to keep them private. Many states have additional laws protecting patients. Again, to the previous question above, is it permissible to not divulge information you know may be a double effect?

Throughout history there have always been ethical issues and choices. In business, law, healthcare, and wartime, there will always be times when an ethical decision needs to be made. The choice that is made may be right or wrong, however, at that time, whoever makes the choice is making it based on the circumstances and information available.

Prior to the 1950s, when bioethics was first being discussed, people making tough decisions didn't think of them as being ethical issues; they probably didn't know what the term was. Today, most people have no real understanding of medical ethics and the decisions they have to make when their loved one is critically ill and dying. It is the job of the healthcare professional to bring out all the options and choices that a family has so that the best decision for that person is made.

Medical ethics will always be around. As technology advances, there will be more choices to make. Take stem cell research. Stem cells are cells that have the potential to become any type of cell. Interest has focused on whether stem cell therapy could alleviate or even cure common degenerative diseases. However, in harvesting these cells they are destructive to an embryo. In taking stem cells, usually the embryo is five to seven days old, so because of this there have been many debates on the ethics of research on early human embryos. Stem cells derived from various sources raise different ethical issues, but their contribution to medical research could be immense. Stem cell research could prove to be the cure for disabling diseases like Alzheimer's, diabetes, and Parkinson's, to name a few. *(McLaren, 2001)* Just like stem cell research, there are legal, moral, and ethical issues when people are frail, elderly, and close to death.

One must know and understand the wishes of that person and what they want. Did they fill out a living will or a do not resuscitate (DNR) form? The question that I always asked families when they started to question what to do when their elderly family member is failing is if you were in this position, if you were the one laying there, what would you want? Asking this question, they usually would respond to be kept comfortable, and by them confirming this question, they usually are at peace with the outcome. When people are in this situation, it gives them time to examine their own moral and belief system.

What kind of medical care would you want if you were too ill or hurt to express your wishes? Advance directives are legal documents that allow you to convey your decisions about end-of-life care ahead of time. They provide a way for you to communicate your wishes to family, friends, and healthcare professionals and to avoid confusion later on. A living will dictates how you feel about care intended to sustain life. You can accept or refuse medical care. There are many issues to address, including the use of dialysis and breathing machines, if you want to be resuscitated if breathing or heartbeat stops, tube feeding, organ or tissue donation. A durable power of attorney for healthcare is a document that names your healthcare proxy, someone you trust to make health decisions if you are unable to do so. It's a lot to think about, but setting up the proper paperwork in the beginning will eliminate a lot of ethical decisions that may have to be made later on. There is a form called the Five Wishes in which you can enter your wish for the person that you want to make decisions for you when you can't. The kind of medical treatment you want. How comfortable do you want to be? How you want people to treat you. What do want your loved ones to know? *(Aging with Dignity, resource section).*

As you can see, there is a lot that family and patients need to think about. Answers are not black and white but gray, and usually not thought about until they are faced with these decisions. No right or wrong answer can be chosen. It is dependent on what disease the person is dealing with and the options of treatments available at that time. Take into consideration how religion and culture factor into this and how much pressure the family puts on that patient, only then does one know if that was the right or wrong decision.

Life is pleasant. Death is peaceful. It's the transition that's troublesome.

— Isaac Asimov

Summary

As you read, aging, death, and dying can be overwhelming. Medical professionals are specialized; there are pulmonologists, cardiologists, orthopedics, neonatologists, gerontologists, and the list go on. These professionals treat a specific disease, so you may have three to six different doctors treating you at the same time depending on what is going on with you. However, it is the end-of-life staff that treats the whole person. They treat not only the body but also the mind and spirit. They understand that treating the whole person helps them in their journey, and that comfort and peace is an ultimate goal that one must achieve.

We live in an age of cultural diversity and global mobility. If you travel back to the dawn of man, they lived in small tribes and took care of their own in sickness and in health. They migrated up from Africa over the landmasses on foot. Today we can get to Australia, Japan, Russia, and Italy in a matter of hours. We leave our birthplace for work and adventure, living our own lives. However, what is different now vs. the distant past and even the recent past is that the care of the sick and dying was by family and friends, not by strangers in residential facilities and nursing homes.

Culture is what defines us. It is our background, ethnicity, and the way we grew up which dictates the way we handle the elderly and ourselves. Remember, America is a multitude of cultures, and even with certain cultures that do carry on the tradition of caring for their elders, the children of that culture do have that opportunity of going off to a college and maybe landing a position in a different state where they get married and have kids of their own. Traditions, although carried on for generations, unfortunately fade over time just because of these factors.

It is important that one understands the process of aging and dying. Remember, aging is a process. As one gets older, the body and organs wear out, just like a machine. Organs slow down and sometimes fail. Bones get frail and break, and the most common bone that breaks in an elderly person is the hip. It is also known that the hip in the elderly as they are walking or just standing can break, causing a fall vs. them falling and breaking a hip. The brain, which is like the mainframe of a computer, atrophies (shrinking, wasting away of the brain cells, due to disease or non-use) so processing memories, experiences, and decisions become much more difficult. As one ages, one is more vulnerable to diseases and illness. Over time these diseases and illnesses wear on the elderly, and then they start going into the dying process.

As we talked in the physiology chapter, the body starts to prepare itself for the final stages of life, evident by the skin being cool to touch, increase in sleep, disorientation to person, place, and time, and incontinence. Urine decreases as the kidneys slow down, congestion develops as the heart starts to slow down, restlessness increases, fluid and food intake decrease, and breathing patterns change. Once the family understands this physical process of dying, there is less panic, and the better off the person is in their process, being more comfortable and peaceful until death.

In the psychosocial-spiritual-mental area of the person that is dying, families and friends will see withdrawal and decreased socialization of that person from them and from reality. The person is more focused now on reflecting back on their life and coming to peace with their eventual end. Patients will have vision-like experiences of seeing past relatives, family members, or friends that have passed on previously. They will be talking out loud to someone and carrying on a normal conversation as if the person were standing there in the room. There have been many instances where in caring for patients I have asked the family who that person is that they are mentioning, and they usually tell me that it is an uncle, aunt, dad, or mom that has already passed.

Giving permission to that person dying is important, not only to them but the family as well. This not only takes the burden and stress off that person and family, it makes their passing more peaceful. Just telling them that it is okay to go, we will be okay, don't worry about things, just focus on your own comfort. Saying things like this to the dying person greatly relieves them, and their passing may actually come quicker. You will most likely see a calmness in that person as they die.

Saying goodbye to that person may sound weird, however it is just like giving permission for them to die. All this helps in the grieving process as the person is dying, and after they pass makes it a much more pleasant experience for family and friends involved. There are a number of ways in which to make this dying process more comfortable—playing soft music that they used to love to listen to, aromatherapy, burning soft scents like lavender or scented candles, as long as they are not too overpowering, bringing in their pet or an animal that they like.

Patients and families all go through overwhelming reactions from the time they find out that they have an incurable disease and their life is limited to the final stage of dying. Remember Kubler-Ross developed five stages to the dying: Denial: (no, not me) of what they were just told. Then anger: (why me)? Bargaining: If you will let me live long enough to do this or that. Depression: They are at the point of realizing that nothing is working, and they are destined to die. Acceptance: The person has come to terms with their own mortality and accepts their fate. Reflective listening is one way to talk with a person that is dying. Acknowledge what they are saying, don't give your opinions, and really listen to what the person is telling you. They are struggling with their life issues and they really want someone to listen to them. In their view this may be the last time they talk or see you, and they so desperately want to share their fears, stories, or whatever it may be with you, so listen to them.

Ethical issues come in with the advent of medical technology, the more that is discovered and the more that doctors can cure illness, the more issues for patients and families to decide what to do. Research companies want to make back their investments, physicians need to continue to see patients so they can charge insurance and Medicare so they can make a living and cover the cost of their office and staff. Nursing homes and residential homes need residents to keep their doors open. So, what does one do? Ethical issues are never black and white. When a person is so weak and loses the ability to swallow, then comes the decision of a feeding tube to keep them alive. When a person's heart or lungs start to give out, do you put the person on a ventilator to keep them alive? There are tough choices. However, if a person has a living will written out, a do not resuscitate (DNR) form filled out, then the person is telling everyone if something happens to me don't resuscitate me and keep me alive by artificial means. One caveat to this is that the POA can overrule these wishes of the patient, and so now comes the ethical dilemma.

The biggest decisions come in when a person wishes to die by physician-assisted suicide or euthanasia. Again, remember this is illegal in all but four states. However, in the coming years more and more states may pass this type of law, so decisions will have to be made by the patient and accepted by the family.

When someone has a debilitating disease and the disease starts to overcome them, like ALS, one choice is palliative sedation, where the patient is sedated so that they don't know or feel what is going on, and this lets the disease take its course until death. A big ethical decision by the patient and family needs to be made here, as the sedation medication will ultimately lead to the person's death. This is where ethics committees come into play, to make sure that the choice by the patient and/or family is the best choice based on the information at the time.

Where do we go from here? Decisions, choices, and documents written out for the wishes of the patient help, but as technology improves, these decisions will not be clear-cut. We all will be part of the older generation someday, and planning will be important not only for you but for your children, so they know what your wishes are. This will make any decisions about your healthcare easier. People are living longer. For the most part, most of us are healthier and better educated and know what we want out of life. We all strive to be healthier so we can live longer, however, the universe can dictate differently. We all are dictated by our genetic makeup, environment, foods we eat, and the lives we lead, but one day we too will face that dreaded decision we never want to think of, and that is our mortality. There is an old saying that the only sure thing is death and taxes. Each year we face taxes and get through it, someday we will face death, and then what?

Exercises/Projects

Below is a list of exercises and projects to consider. Life comes and goes so fast that being prepared can alleviate a lot of stress. Choose one or two or do them all. These are here for you to think about your life and how you would handle your own death.

Your ideal and/or probable death: Think about this. If you had a choice in how you would die, what would it be? Where would you want to be? Write it out. You may be surprised.

Write out a letter of goodbye. Add what you will miss, what you regret not doing, wish you had done, people you wanted to see and didn't. Include the joy you had through your life, what you cherish the most. If you can do it all over again, what would you change, if anything?

Think about what your ideal funeral would be. Would you have a service, burial, or cremation? What would you want your family to do, have a party, or be somber and mourn?

If you had a debilitating disease like ALS, Parkinson's, or cancer, and you knew what lies ahead, would you want physician-assisted suicide or euthanasia as an option?

Write out your will. What do you want to leave to whom? Also, write out your wishes. Who do you want to make decisions for you when you can't? What kind of medical treatment do you want or don't want?

For this exercise you will need to be in a quiet place in your mind. Make the room dark, play some quiet, peaceful music, light a scented candle (if you so desire). Be at peace with your mind. Close your eyes and let yourself go to a peaceful place that you have experienced in the past (a sandy beach, a forest—you should be alone in this area). Feel the breeze, the sun on your face, and the warmth of the day. Imagine you have died and this was your heaven. Who would you want to be there with you, your family, pets, and friends? Bring that person there with you in your mind. Talk to whoever is there to express your joys, sorrows, things that you love and miss. Walk with them on that beach or path in the forest or wherever you are. Feel this in your mind and heart and let your emotions go. Once you are back in the real world, write down what you felt. If you want to share this, you can, or you can keep this private; it is up to you.

Resources

1. National Hospice and Palliative Care Organization: www. nhpco.org/research.
2. Aging with Dignity, P.O. Box 1661, Tallahassee, Florida 32302-1661. www.agingwithdignity.org
3. Barbara Karnes, P.O. Box 822139, Vancouver, WA 98682. www.bkbooks.com
4. Center for Medicare & Medicaid Services. www.medicare. gov (800-633-4227)
5. Office of Inspector General, US Department of Health and Human Services. www.oig.hhs.gov
6. American Medical Association. www.ama-assn.org
7. Arizona Hospice and Palliative Organization. www.ahpco. org (each state should have their own organization separate from the national organization)
8. American Geriatric Society. www.americangeriatrics.org
9. Compassion and Choices. www.compassionandchoices.org
10. National Institute of Neurological Disorders and Stroke. www.ninds.nih.gov
11. Alzheimer's Association. www.alz.org

References

Anka, Paul. "My Way." 1969. Concord Records.

Ember, Carol R. & Ember, Melvin. *Cultural Anthropology*, Sixth Edition. Chapter 2, Cultural Variations. Prentice Hall, 1990.

Matteson, Mary Ann & McConnell, Eleanor S. *Gerontological Nursing: Concepts and Practice.* W.B. Saunders Co. Philadelphia, PA. 1988 (ch. 5, 16, 17).

Mosby's Dictionary of Medicine, Nursing & Health Professions. 9th ed. Mosby, Elsevier Inc. 2013.

Berkowitz, Aaron. M.D., PhD, *Clinical Pathophysiology.* MedMaster, Inc. 2007.

Karnes, Barbara, RN, *Gone From My Sight: The Dying Experience.* 2009.

Durham, Eileen, BSN, RN and Weiss, Leslie, MA, BSN, RN. "How Patients Die." American Journal of Nursing, vol. 97, no. 12, December 1997.

Bell, Whitley Karen. *Living at the End of Life.* Sterling Ethos, New York. 2010.

Kleinman, Paul. *Psych 101, A Crash Course in the Science of the Mind.* Adams Media, MA. 2012.

Kubler-Ross, Elisabeth, MD. *On Death and Dying,* Scribner, Simon & Schuster, NY. 1969.

Kubler-Ross, Elisabeth. *Questions & Answers on Death and Dying, A Companion Volume to On Death and Dying.* A Touchstone Book, by Simon & Schuster, 1997.

Lane, Lara Lynn. .” *Gale Encyclopedia of Psychology*. 2005.

American Heritage Medical Dictionary. Houghton, Mifflin Harcourt. 2008.

The Stanford Encyclopedia of Philosophy. The Metaphysics Research Lab Center for the Study of Language and Information, Stanford University, Stanford, CA. 94305. 2013

Hallenbeck, Terri. “Vermont Governor Signs End-Of-Life Bill.” *The Burlington Vt. Free Press*. 5/20/2013

Journal American Medical Association: Palliative Sedation: Erin Brender, MD; Alison Burke, MA; Richard M. Glass, MD. JAMA. 2005; 294(14): 1850. doi:10.1001/jama.294.14.1850.

Source: National Hospice and Palliative Care Organization.

For additional information, please download NHPCO’s Facts &Figures on Hospice from the Web site: www.nhpco.org/research.

National Hospice and Palliative Care Organization, New Hospice facts & figures. For Immediate Release: January 11, 2012. “Dying Americans Using Hospice Care Remains Stable but New Report Reveals Drop in Length of Service.”

Kubler-Ross, Elisabeth & Kessler, David. *On Grief and Grieving, Finding the Meaning of Grief Through the Five Stages of Loss*. Published by Scribner NY, New York. 2005.

Cooper, Phyllis G., RN, MN, and McKesson, HBOC Clinical Reference Systems. McKesson LLC. 2001

Worden’s, William J. *Grief Counseling and Grief Therapy*. 4th edition, Springer. 2008.

Karnes, Barbara, RN. *My Friend, I Care: The Grief Experience*. 2009.

Holland, Debra MS, PhD. *The Essential Guide to Grief and Grieving: An Understanding Guide to Coping with Loss and Finding Hope and Meaning Beyond*. Penguin Group NY, NY 2011

Murray Beckmann, Ruth; Zentner Proctor, Judith; Yakimo, Richard. *Health Promotion Strategies Through the Life Span.* 8th ed. Ch. 7, Spiritual and Religious Influences. Ch. 17, Dying and Death: The Last Developmental Stage. Pearson Prentice Hall, 2009.

Singer, Peter. *Practical Ethics*, third edition. Cambridge University Press, 2011.

Levine, Carol. *Taking Sides: Clashing Views on Controversial Bioethical Issues.* 5th edition. The Dushkin Publishing Group, Inc. 1993.

Panza, Christopher, PhD; Potthast, Adam, PhD. *Ethics for Dummies*, Ch 12: Dealing with Mad Scientist: Biomedical Ethics. Wiley's Publishing, Inc. 2010.

American Medical Association, Code of Medical Ethics. http://www.ama-assn.org/ama/pub/physician-resources/medical-ethics/code-medical-ethics.page www.ama-assn.org/ama/pub/.../medical-ethics/code-medical-ethics

American Hospital Association. *The Patients' Bill of Rights* AHA, Chapter 6: Right Truths and Consents. Section 4. Readings. Copyright Philip A Pecorino 2002.

American Nurses Association, Code of Ethics for Nurses. 1985.

McLaren, Anne. "Ethical and Social Considerations of Stem Cell Research." Nature, 414, 129-131 (1 November 2001) | doi:10.1038/35102194

Review Requested:

We'd like to know if you enjoyed the book.
Please consider leaving a review on the platform
from which you purchased the book.